I Lost 100 Pounds and You Can Too!

My Harrowing Weight Loss Journey

By Carol Langkamp

Part One

2015

TABLE OF CONTENTS

THE BEGINNING:

Inspiration and Motivation

When I decided to write this book about my weight loss journey, I thought it would be easy. How hard could it be? I began the writing process by sifting through my Facebook page and collecting posts specific to this journey.

Once I started this mission, I discovered I had lots of pictures and inspiring messages that I found while carousing online. There were more motivational notes than writings centered on my weight struggles. Therefore, I decided to write a little about the importance of your attitude along the way.

Let me give you a little history here. When I first started this mission, I weighed my heaviest ever. Just like the pig that ate too many donuts in the children's story. I hate to share this number, as it felt like I had ballooned overnight! I topped out at 334 pounds! Never, ever did I believe I would reach that extreme weight. The scale seemed to stare me in the face. I thought, "How on Earth did I ever get here?" Yet, the truth was, I had arrived—all 300 and 34 pounds of me. At first, I could not remember what year I first saw this immense weight but then realized it was the year 2004. Thankfully I can share with you the fact that I am nowhere close to that weight today. I weighed in last week at 238.4 pounds!

When I first started this journey, I was ready to give up on life. I was employed, but was not happy with my job, did not have many friends, and just could not find a way to get out of this dreadful situation. My living situation was dependent on family since I lived with my older sister. My sisters and the rest of my family did not understand or support me in most of my decisions. Just like the rest of my life, I hid my feelings with food, stuffed the emotions down, and got rid of them. The problem was I became increasingly bigger and also more and more depressed. Something had to give.

Therefore, I started on yet another weight loss plan but this one was a program through O.S.U. medical center. Perhaps I could find the solution to my struggles. I started a therapy-based program that addressed my binge eating disorder and my personal issues. With the help of a therapist, I planned out personal weight loss strategies, down to what groceries I needed and when I would start the program. Dr. Phil McGraw had just come out with his weight loss plan and I decided I would start the first of February 2004. I watched the television show faithfully and could not believe all the success stories. My Dad and I had some heart-to-heart conversations via email and telephone and he was so supportive of my decisions. In one of his emails he encouraged me to make the necessary changes and wrote:

> *"I think you should concentrate on the positive WHAT IFS. What would it be like to wear a size 14 dress? How would you like to run around the block? How about a two piece bathing suit? It seems that those who have succeeded in reaching their goals feel like a new person and literally start a new life."*

In yet another of his emails he wrote a superbly profound question to me:

> *"What if tomorrow doesn't come??WHEN IS THE RIGHT TIME??....Have you ever dreamed of WHAT IT WOULD BE LIKE?"*

Inspiration and motivation are the real keys to success. Find it, live it, and be it. The days that I struggle the most are the days that my Facebook page is flooded with inspirational quotes, pictures, stories, and comments. There are times when I think I may have scared everyone away because of my serial posting. However, I need these posts and believe if they help me, then they probably can help someone else too. It is important to fill your tank with optimism. These inspirational posts help me find support as well as find my inner strength and power to survive. This helps me remember to break down each day and focus on just one smaller unit of time; such as a minute, hour, meal, morning, evening or day. Doing this helps me succeed and meet my goals.

I must tell you that before starting any weight loss or exercise plan, you should consult your physician. Believe me, my doctors have discussed my weight with me over and over again and finally I am educating *them* about what works for me!

REALITY SETS IN

The Big Girls Club?!

Truthfully, this journey started back in my childhood but I am going to begin this chapter in the middle of the voyage. I hope it doesn't confuse you too much.

Twelve years ago, I found myself depressed, at my heaviest weight ever, and desperately seeking help to find a way out of this downward spiral. I met with a therapist who helped me prepare for the journey. Part of the reason for my therapy was that I had an ailing father I was worried about and both my parents lived in my childhood home in New York which is quite a distance from where I live. My counselor worked with me to devise shopping lists and weekly meal plans. She met with me every week to assist in coping with emotional stress. We both decided on the start day of this journey as the first of February. I would be following Dr. Phil's Weight Loss Program. This plan was simple for me to follow and I was pleasantly surprised that I did not feel hungry and also that the weight came off fairly quickly. At this point, I had not added a key component of weight loss–the dreaded exercise. However without the help of exercising, in a little over two months I was down from 330 pounds to 280 pounds. I hit that the very morning my Dad passed away. I had just made it to 50 pounds lost. This was obviously a very meaningful time for me as you will see.

I told my Dad I wanted to lose at least 50 pounds and he had to be there when I made it that far. He was admitted to the hospital on April Fool's Day that year with a fatal pulmonary disease. The last few weeks of my Dad's life, were some of the precious but few times I ever saw my Dad cry. He was so proud of me and bragged to everyone that came in his room. He also was my most supportive and biggest cheerleader in my weight loss pursuits. Unfortunately, he died before I made it to my ideal weight, but at least he saw me within a few pounds of losing fifty. I know he was with me when I got on the scale and hit the 50-pound loss mark. I loved having Dad so proud of me and having him share in my milestone made me feel very good.

The grief was traumatic to me and depression soon set in. Unfortunately some of my days were also filled with regret about the poor relation I had with my Dad most of my life as well as some family issues that popped up the last day of my dad's life. Part of my problem was insomnia which became so extreme that I asked my Doctor for sleeping pills. It was during this time though that I found a new passion, one I never ever thought I would have. I started taking ballroom dance lessons and once again found some happiness in life. Through the movement of dance I found I could forget about my insecurities, fears, worries and problems and enjoy the music and the dance.

However, my weight crept back up and so did some health issues along with it. I found out I had arthritis and severe cartilage loss in both my knees due to my weight. Even with these issues, I kept dancing whenever I could and found the dance studio became my second home. It was a place that I received love, encouragement, and support—things I direly needed.

ADDICTIONS

Another truth emerges

Several years later, I found myself still struggling and decided to go to Overeaters Anonymous or OA. At this point, I did not realize as I do now, that I was a food addict. If you do not understand what this means, it is similar to being a drug addict. Instead of being hooked on drugs, I'm hooked on sugar-filled foods. Sit me down next to a one-pound bag of M&Ms and you might be surprised how quickly those little 'melt in your mouth' candies disappear.

It was at this time that I realized this problem with my eating was more than I could handle on my own. I needed help and turned to OA for support, thinking it would be an easy task. My insecurities ran wild during the meetings. I felt like I couldn't share or speak up. And, I was petrified of reaching out to someone. What would they think of me? Time went on and after about a month, I was advised to choose someone to sponsor me for the program. Ugh! I needed to face reality? "No!" my inner voices screamed.

I tried a few sponsors but each time I felt the person did not click with me or felt they did not understand my situation well enough to help. The truth is my insecurities came out to play once again and I put my blinders on so I would not have to face change. Therefore, I stopped going to the meetings but over the years have revisited them as well as some other groups that deal with Binge Eating Disorder and Compulsive Overeating.

I really do truly understand addictive behavior, being out of control, feeling powerless and the nonstop, mindless eating without any end in sight. There are some realizations I found out about addictions and this is not just for food addicts but crosses all the boundaries of addictions. Additionally, I understand a variety of addictions as I once dated a sex addict, and also found I could have fallen into the traps of alcoholism if I had not seriously thought about the consequences.

Addictions do not truly bring you what you are looking for. You are looking for happiness and the desire to be loved. The only way to do that, folks, is to love yourself and let go of all your fears. Move past these fears. Look outside of yourself and see what the world has to offer, what God has to offer you. There is so much more to life than drugs, alcohol, and food. They do not fill the void. There is nothing that compares to being loved, and being happy. Money cannot buy you love. Money cannot buy you happiness. True happiness starts from within and radiates outward. Self-love and acceptance are the keys to breaking through and having a fulfilling life.

One of the ways I have found to work on my self is by looking in the mirror and telling myself I love you. It may seem corny at first but after the initial week or so, it becomes real. Also, I have self-affirmations posted all over my apartment, and even have some positive statements written on the bathroom mirror. These are all reminders that I am worthwhile and deserve to be happy and fulfilled.

NOURISHING YOUR BODY

Food plan for your entire life!

Some people think that they're deprived when they go on a food plan. However, I have found, that if you develop a food plan that will work with you throughout your entire life, you won't deprive yourself. You may be making different food choices than you're accustomed to, but you are not being deprived. For example, the food plan that I am currently using is a 24-day plan. Part of that plan is using protein powder or meal replacement shakes mixed with almond milk. Sometimes I also add ice cubes since this makes a really frothy milkshake that is delicious. In fact, I love this milkshake and it tastes magnificent. I am treating myself with this yummy milkshake. Just think about it, you are not depriving yourself when you take care of yourself. It is the complete opposite because you have deprived yourself of living a wonderful life and being able to enhance that life with a balanced healthy lifestyle. You will probably find you have more joy in your life too as you have more energy and feel better about yourself.

BALANCED LIVING

What is that?

Living a balanced life means balancing the amount of sleep, social time, work time and personal time throughout your day. There are a variety of questions one should reflect on when checking the balance of your life.

Is my food plan nutritionally balanced? How about my life and the way I live it? Am I getting enough work done or am I too involved in social events, playing computer games, FB, or email? Do I give myself time to regroup my emotions when needed and reset myself for contentment and peace? Also, am I getting a good quality sleep at night and enough sleep on a regular basis?

Here is what I have learned about balance and the way it equates to life. Life is not about 100% perfection. Balance is a mishmash of everyday living where sometimes you are equal on both sides, sometimes you are way out of whack and other times you are pretty damn close. It is the times when things are off balance or off kilter that are crucial lessons in life. For example, have you ever found yourself in a very stressful situation and thought you would not be able to survive? After surviving what seemed to be something so awful, you can now reflect on the things that you learned and how this event made you stronger.

More important to me than balancing my life is gratitude. Start each and every day being grateful for what you have, even if the only thing you can think of is that you have your whole body including all your senses. There are a multitude of things to be grateful about and sometimes we forget them. I know this is really simplistic but remember to enjoy life and be thankful!

WHAT IS IMPORTANT THEN?

Why does this matter?

Life is not about how many possessions you have or how much money you make, even though most people seem to think that way. It is about taking care of you. You are number one, not your rich neighbors or friends.

You need to take care of your health. Make that your number one priority. You are given one life and only one life. Don't let anybody fool you. Humans are not cats so they don't have nine lives. You've only got one life. It's not a dress rehearsal or a game. It is life. You need to live it to the fullest, no matter what. Make the best of your day.

Here is a good example of this illusion for you. In the past, most people looked up to Donald Trump and thought he had it made in life and was so successful. Look at him now. He is in politics, supposedly. He's class clown of the world. People are making fun of him left and right. Who wants that? And besides, obviously money isn't happiness, so go and live your life. Go for the natural highs that are abundant in life. That's what really counts. *Lift* your dreams higher. I admit the first time I wrote this it was a typo, but then I decided I like the word lift instead of live. Live your dreams, take risks. Fulfill your worthiness.

REALITY CHECK

Bumps in the road

It's time for a new message. Yesterday, I fell off the wagon. It was an emotional roller coaster. I shed some tears. I actually threw in the towel and said, "Screw it! I'm gonna eat what I am gonna eat!" I ate horribly and was ready to deal with the consequences. I reached out to several people, but for the most part, nobody was available. After two hours, though, my trainer got back to me and I had a heart-to-heart talk with him. I know that he says he is hesitant to reach out to me at these times because he feels that I need to do this on my own. But I get a lot of value from the conversations that I have with him, it opens my eyes to many things especially when I have slipped back to the point where my blinders are on and I can't see my success. Part of my eating disorder and my deeply critical thinking is down the track of feeling like a failure and being worthless.

Those are all freaking lies! The more I learn, the more I grow, the more weight I lose, the better person I become and the more I realize those statements are untrue. Don't fool yourself into believing them. Don't go down that road. You have a choice. You want to live? GO OUT AND LIVE IT! Don't sit there and let that wound fester and turn into something that it was never meant to be. You can sit there and wallow in pity and negativity. Or, you can say, "World, you know what? It is time to shut these bad habits down! It is time to get out there! It is time to learn. It is time to be what I am truly meant to be."

Even at almost a 100-pound weight loss, there are still lessons to be learned. Most of my life has been spent mindlessly eating. I learned it year in, year out for so many years that it is almost a more comfortable option for me than eating healthy. It is the difference of 45 years of unhealthy habits to about 3 years of healthier habits. It is so important to take care of me by making a pact to eat healthy all day long. I take it one step at a time, one minute at a time, one hour at a time and one day at a time. Also, I take care of myself by exercising on a daily basis. I have found this to be a total mood changer for me and research shows this is a reality. Why fight something that works well and helps get you to your goals, right?

Recently, I came across "The Strength Camp Challenge." In my heart, I want to be part of it. I wish I had found it earlier so I could try it this year. However, I don't think my body is strong enough yet. Plus you really have to train for this kind of competition and build up your strength and stamina.

Next year is coming, and you watch, I will be part of that challenge. I will be there and I will compete. Yeah! I like the limelight. I will admit it. I may be shy at times and I may not feel like it, but I love to compete. It's not so much the competition against others, the awards, or the recognition. These are great incentives, but it is more about competing against myself. I want to do better each time I walk into the gym, dance floor, and any other walk of life. If I can do a better job than I did the last time, then I can take pride in how far I have come.

I was talking about having blinders on earlier and I wanted to share a realization. I couldn't see. I couldn't see how far I've come. I really seriously did not know how far I had come. That's why it's so important to have the people in my life that help me break down those walls. I really feel that those blockers are part of that negative voice inside me telling me I am worthless and invaluable.

However, I put the brakes on and I got a new message inside of me. It says:

"World, watch out, 'cause this girl's worth so much and going far!"

Now, it is your turn. I want to reach out to you and share a reality with you. No matter how you feel right now, right this very moment, please listen to my message. You are on this Earth for a reason. You are here. Anybody that is here on this Earth is worthwhile. You deserve to be whole! Do not live your life as a half. You want to be whole and you deserve to be whole. Whole feels so much better and is so much healthier.

THE GOLDEN KEY

Self Doubt Strikes Again

Remember when you were a little kid riding a carousel and you could reach out for the golden key which would get you a ride for free? Somehow in life people are always trying to find their golden key, which is an easier route to reaching a goal or attaining what they really want to in their life. For me, I am still searching for that golden key as I still am consumed with looking for a better food plan or easier way to get to my final goal.

The closer I get to my goal weight, the harder this journey becomes. I am still riddled with self-doubt and still fall prey to my binge eating disorder. There are times when I have so much insecurity, so little energy and so many problems focusing my attention on anything that is important. My emotions run wild and I let the scared little girl inside, take over my life.

The road that I am on now is uncertain and I'm unsure of my future. Nothing is the same which makes me uncomfortable. However, I know I am in the driver's seat and maintain control. It is up to me to make the choice and keep going. It may be difficult at times but remember to look how far you have come. Do not give up. You are so close to breaking through.

I Lost 100 Pounds and You Can Too!

It is times like these when I have changed the way I look at things. Children somehow experience joys in life without all this analysis and prejudgment. Therefore, I have found if I live my life through the eyes and wonder of a child, it really helps.

For example, I went to the holiday light show at the zoo all by myself. Normally, this would depress me because of being alone. However, I decided in my mind, to try and experience these lights as if I was a young child seeing them for the first time. It made me enjoy them so much more than I would have normally. Another time, I was at a corn maze hunting for animal pictures that were hidden along the pathway. My friend was surprised when I started calling and yelling to the animals for help finding them.

My point is that it is very important to look at yourself and live your life in a positive light. Make it fun and exciting. There is not really a golden key so just stick fast to the way that works the best for you.

CONCLUSION

The End Of The Journey?

I need to somehow conclude this book that I have written. I want to say something about how I consider this a weight loss journey. However, when you think about a journey you think about an ending. Well, much to my astonishment, I have realized and discovered that there is no end to this journey. When I try to end it, I go back to my old habits of binge eating the stuff that does not nourish my body. It really does not matter what diet you try, but you will find that any diet will work only for a short time if you view it as a short term goal. And each kind of diet will work for some people but not for every single person.

The key to a food plan is finding the right one that works for you. It may take some trial and error sometimes–meaning you need to try some things out, and give it an honest chance. Be truthful with yourself–are you following the plan wholeheartedly or are you cheating yourself and lying about it? Yes, obviously I am very familiar with this method and have done it myself. However, if you really want change to occur, you need to put your whole heart into it with 100% commitment. Pick a plan that you feel is doable, and commit to doing it for a month. Consider it a trial period if that helps. It takes 21 days to change a habit. If after the trial period of 21 to 30 days you still feel it's not working for you, then, by all means, try something else. The important thing is that you do not give up. Do not decide this is the end. In this battle, the only end is death and that is futile. Keep moving forward to your goal.

Be careful of the words you choose to use, the way you think, your actions, your thoughts, and your ideas on this journey. These are all relevant as it is not just about eating a certain way and exercising. It is about your mindset and your attitude. It's about living and risk taking as well as going outside your comfort zone and stretching yourself beyond the boundaries that you are accustomed to. Go for it! You can do it. I did and I guarantee if you are reading this now, you have it in you to make a change. What is holding you back?

Remember the road may be winding, it may be bumpy, and it may be crazy at times. If you fall off, get back on that road and keep going. You can do this. Believe in yourself! Remember your dreams. You got this! Now, go out and conquer the world!

Carol Langkamp

"inside me there is a voice that just won't let go….

inside me there's a dream that just won't give up…

inside me… i'm discovering the freedom to fly

the strength within myself,

carries me high, toward my destiny"

Seasons of The Heart © 1993 Curtis Allen
Vandevander

I Lost 100 Pounds and You Can Too!

About the Author

Carol Langkamp lives in Columbus, Ohio. She enjoys tutoring, singing, dancing, biking, walking, wildlife, travel, and Zumba. She aspires to be a world-class Zumba instructor. This is her first book and she treasures it dearly.

If you would like to help her out, she would really appreciate your feedback on this book. Please leave a review at Amazon.com.

Also, if you would like to read more about her weight loss journey, you can follow her at this blog address: cllsblogs.blogspot.com.

Thanks!

Special Thanks

Mom, I am so glad to be able to share this journey with you. My next goal is for you to see me under 200! Dad, even though you are in heaven, I want to thank you so much for all those encouraging words, the praise and even the challenges you gave me. I admit I am still working on one right now. Thanks so much for cheering me on, I can still hear you cheering from heaven! I love and miss you!

Also, I need to thank my siblings and their families. I know at times I have been difficult and not easy to live with. Thanks for supporting me in those moments and throughout the years. I am very grateful to you and really appreciate all your help and support.

This book would not have come to fruition without loads of help from my dear friend, Dale Roberts, who is like a brother to me. I don't know if he realizes that or not. Thank you for all the time, support and dedication that you have given to me over the years. I really appreciate all that you have done. Kelli, thanks for sharing in this process, coming up with the title and all your support and help throughout as well as your friendship too.

To my friends, far and wide: Thanks so much for supporting me, encouraging me, praising me and cheering me on during this journey. Unfortunately, I am not finished yet so I hope you are not tired of my Facebook posts.

Lastly, a big part of my life the last two years or so has been my dedication to my training. Keith Oliver, my "Biggest Loser" trainer, is awesome and does an excellent job with an encouraging word when it's needed and a challenge now and then too. If you're ever in Delaware, Ohio and want a great trainer, I suggest you look him up. He has become a dear friend to me, a true supporter and he's helped me out of some very troublesome times. He is part of the reason why I have lost more than fifty pounds just this last year. Keith, I couldn't have made it this far without you. You are worth your weight in gold!

Somehow, I am not done yet. I need to acknowledge my God, who put the right people in my life at the right times. I am so grateful for my life and the abundance within it.

www.ingramcontent.com/pod-product-compliance
Lightning Source LLC
Chambersburg PA
CBHW061941280526
45787CB00004B/1685